D1608793

THE BRAIN

BODYWORKS

Tracy Maurer

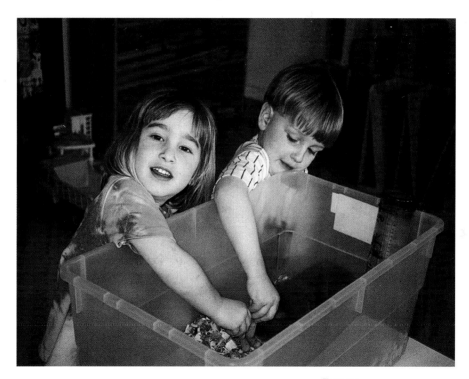

The Rourke Corporation, Inc.
Vero Beach, Florida 32964

Tracy M. Maurer specializes in non-fiction and business writing. Her most recently published children's books include the Let's Dance Series, also from Rourke Publishing.

With appreciation to Lois M. Nelson, Paige Henson, Steven and Linda Dingman, Brittany Morrison, Beverly Dunn, Dr. Rosemary Jackson - Georgia College and State University, the Jewish Community Center School, Milwaukee, WI, and Northside Elementary School, Milledgeville, GA.

PHOTO CREDITS:
© Linda A. Dingman: title page, pages 10, 12, 13; © Timothy L. Vacula: cover, pages 8, 17, 21; © Lois M. Nelson: page 7, 18; © Diane Farleo: page 15

ILLUSTRATION: © Todd Tennyson: page 4

EDITORIAL SERVICES: Janice L. Smith for Penworthy Learning Systems

CREATIVE SERVICES: East Coast Studios, Merritt Island, Florida

Library of Congress Cataloging-in-Publication Data

Maurer, Tracy, 1965-
    The brain / by Tracy Maurer.
        p. cm. — (Bodyworks)
    Summary: Describes the parts of the brain and how they function to control the body and provide personality and memory.
        ISBN 0-86593-585-8
    1. Brain Juvenile literature. [1. Brain.] I. Title. II. Series: Maurer, Tracy, 1965- Bodyworks.
QP376.M386 1999
612.8'2—dc21   99-23388
                                                                CIP

Printed in the USA

TABLE OF CONTENTS

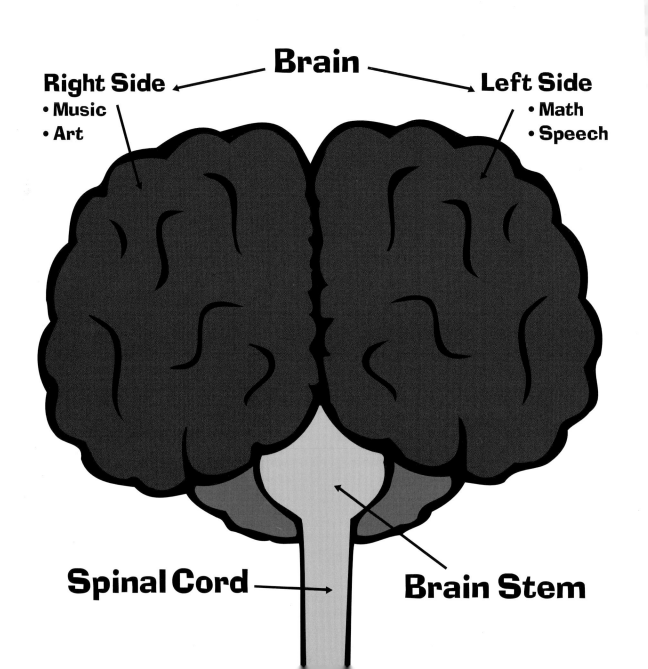

Brain

Right Side
• Music
• Art

Left Side
• Math
• Speech

Spinal Cord

Brain Stem

YOU ARE YOUR BRAIN

Your brain controls who you are. No other brain works exactly like yours. The gray, noodle-like layer called the **cortex** (KAWR TEKS) holds your personality. You talk, feel, move, think, learn, and remember like no one else.

The brain stem tucks up into the brain's gray matter. It forms a bump at the top of the **spinal cord** (SPY nul KORD). The brain stem helps control your lungs and heart rate. It oversees other jobs that keep you alive.

The brain stem forms a bump at the top of the spinal cord.

THE SIGNAL CENTER

Nerves all over your body send signals to the spinal cord and the brain. They send news about the world outside. Nerves tell the brain what's happening inside your body, too.

The brain uses special **brain cells** (BRAYN SELZ) to understand the signals. If the brain wants you to act, it flashes back new signals. These travel along 47 miles (76 kilometers) of nerves. For example, your brain may tell your fingers' nerves to turn the page now.

The brain gets billions of signals at once. What signals do you think are going to this girl's brain?

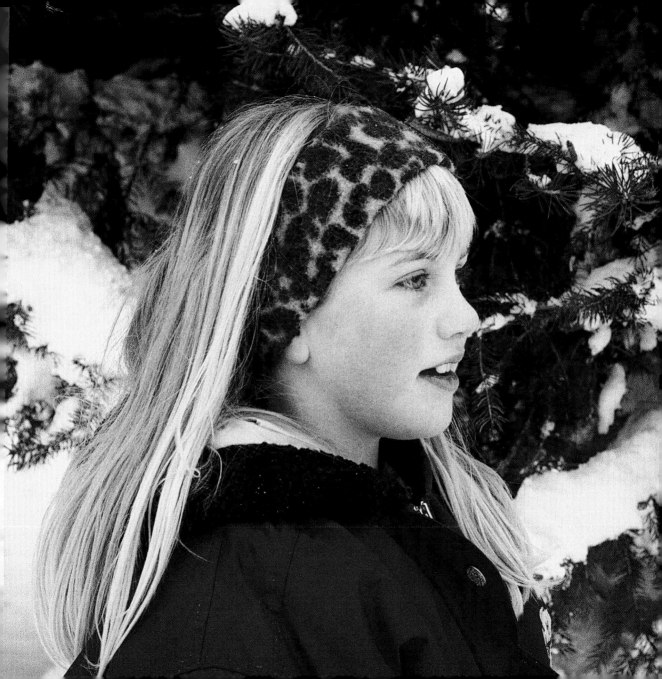

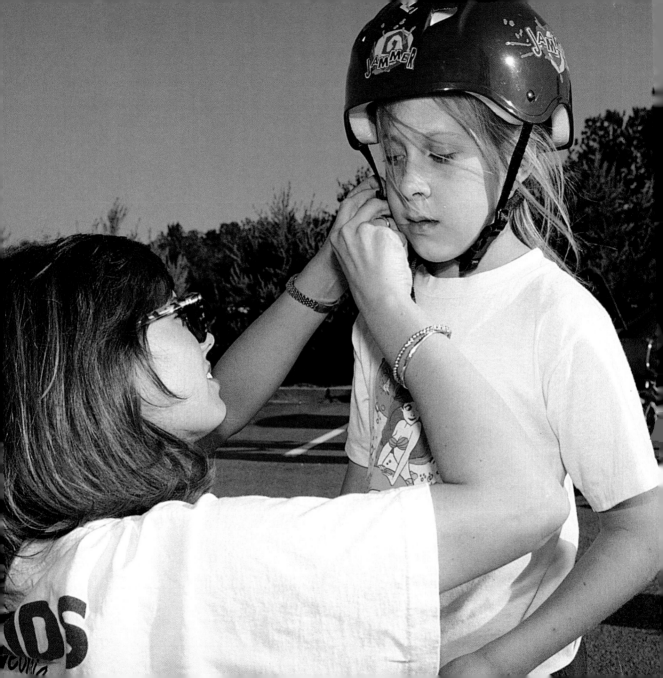

YOUR HARDHAT

Rub your head. Can you feel hard, bumpy skull bones? They fit together like a curved jigsaw puzzle. These bones make a hardhat that protects your brain. The brain floats in **liquid** (LIK wid) that pads it. Wearing a bike helmet adds padding if you hit your head.

You protect your brain by never **abusing** (uh BYOOZ ing) alcohol or drugs. Such abuse kills brain cells. You have billions of brain cells at birth. You never get new ones. Once brain cells die, they are gone forever.

The skull protects the brain. A helmet adds an extra layer of padding.

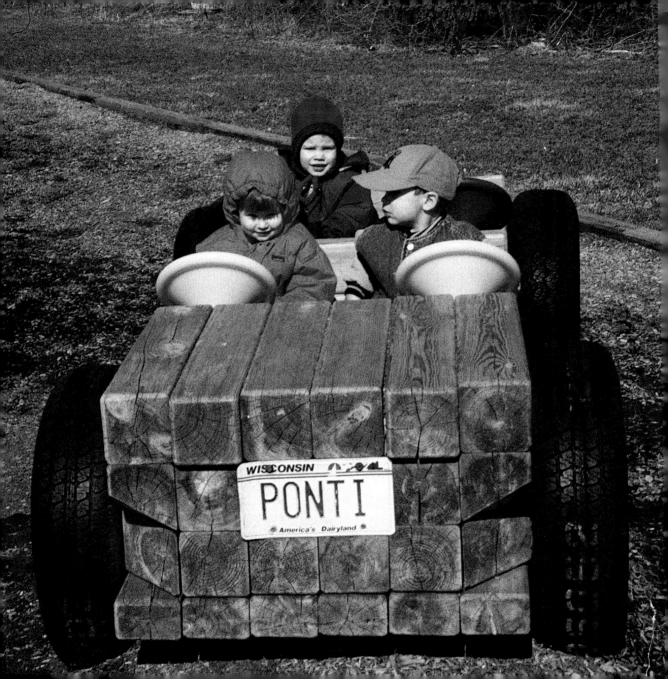

THE BRAIN NEVER SLEEPS

You spend about one-third of your life sleeping. Your brain never takes a break, however. It constantly checks everything your body does. Even when you sleep, your brain stays active.

Dreams come from your brain. Sometimes the brain uses more energy at night than during the day. Dreams may help people deal with daytime events. Even bad dreams may be good.

At night, your brain makes dreams.
When you play in the daytime,
your brain lets you pretend.

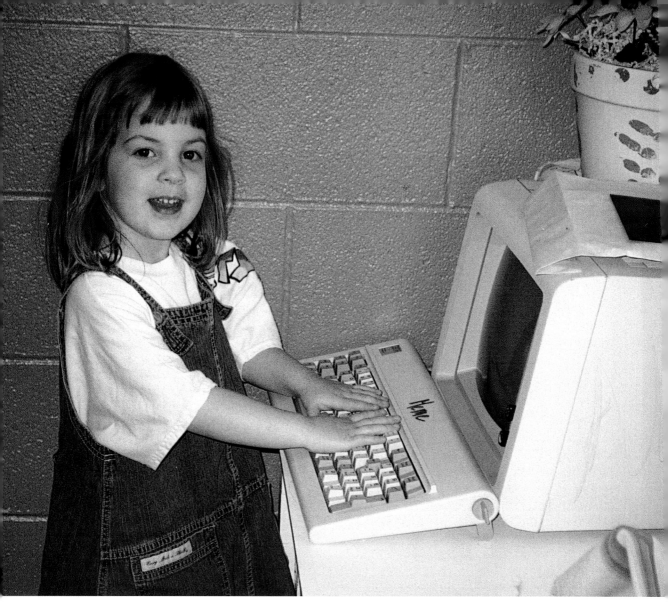

The brain can do more tasks than the most advanced computer.

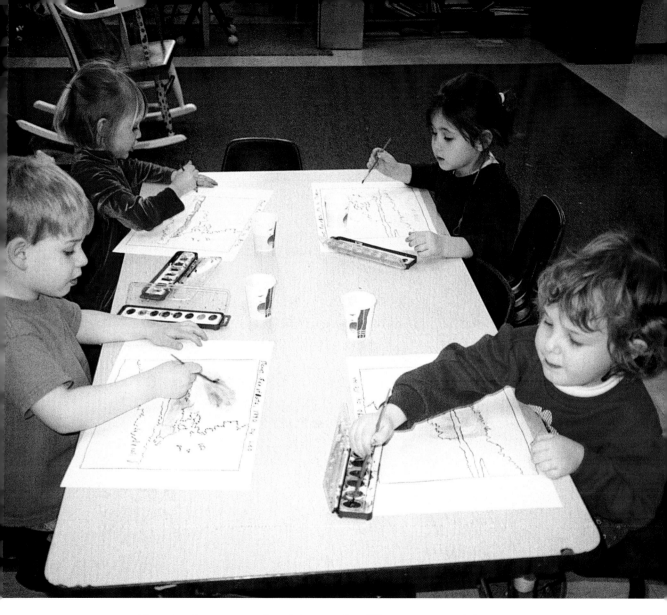

Your brain stores what it learns in different parts of the cortex.

LEFT AND RIGHT THINKING

The brain has two sides. Each controls the opposite side of the body. Your left side tells your right arm to wave. A bridge of cells helps each side know what the other is doing. That's why you can clap your hands.

Each side also controls certain skills. The right side deals with music and other art forms. The left side handles numbers, problem solving, and words. Sometimes the center for words grows in the right side instead of the usual left. When this happens a person is left-handed.

The right side of the brain can show ideas by drawing or painting.

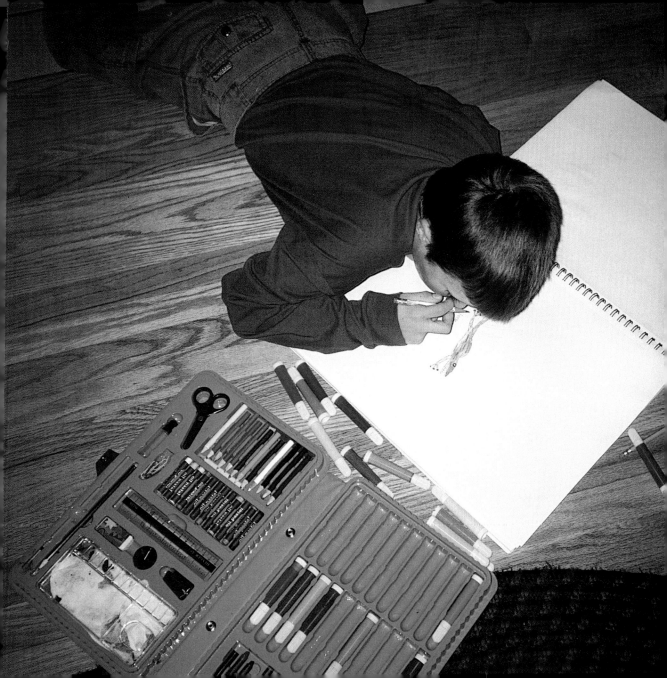

PAIN STOPPERS

If you cut yourself, nerves send the news to your brain. The brain reads these signals as pain. The brain may send out natural painkillers called **endorphins** (en DAWR finz). These **chemicals** (KEM i kulz) quiet the nerves and slow the flow of pain signals.

Endorphins may be sent out at other times. A rush of them after a long run makes a jogger feel happy. Scientists learn about chemicals like these all the time. These chemicals help unlock the brain's secrets.

The brain reads pain signals sent from wounds. The brain itself does not feel very much pain.

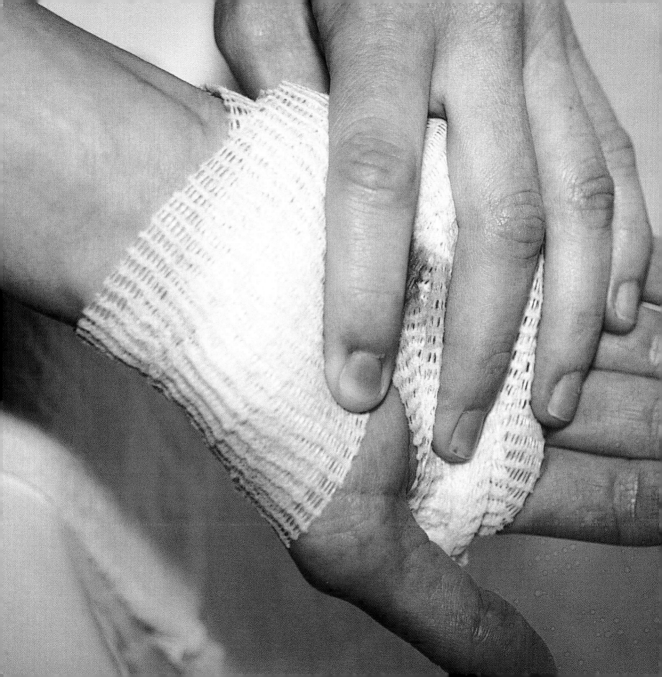

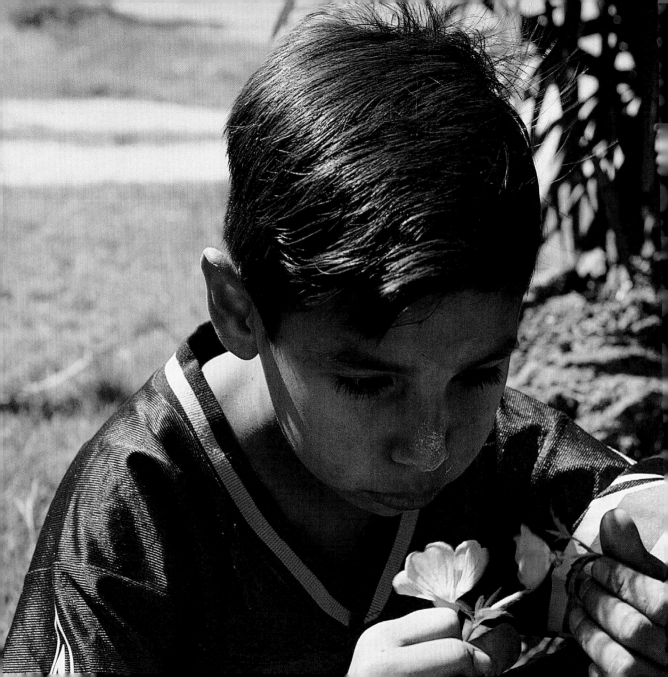

THE MIND MATTERS

The lower brain controls skills. It tells your hand how to hold a pencil and how to write numbers. Your higher brain, or **mind** (MYND), lets you think. It gives you ideas to write or talk about.

The mind makes humans different from other animals. It lets people hope, ask questions, think, and believe. It makes them want to reach a goal. Sometimes sick people believe they will get better, and they do!

Scientists study the brain to learn its amazing powers. Even their curiosity about the brain comes from their minds.

The mind makes it possible to see, smell, and feel.

HOPE FOR A CURE

The spinal cord starts at the brain's base. It continues all the way down the backbone. Every signal to and from the brain runs on this pencil-thick cord.

The spinal cord can be cut or hurt. Then the brain may not be able to tell the body to move. The body cannot tell the brain what it feels. A person may become **paralyzed** (PAIR uh lyzd) or may even die. Every year about 8,000 people hurt their spinal cords. Many must use wheelchairs to move. Remember, their minds still work! Doctors hope to cure hurt spinal cords some day.

People in wheelchairs go to school and play with friends. They use wheelchairs instead of legs to move.

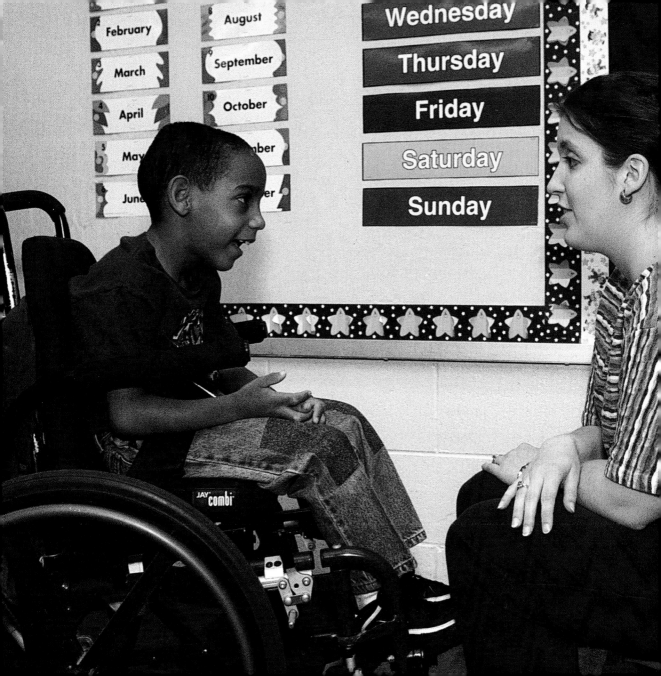

BRAIN FOOD

The body breaks food down into **nutrients** (NOO tree ents). Some nutrients mix with the brain's chemicals. This mix may change how you feel. Eating sugar can make you feel very excited. Drinking warm milk can make you feel tired.

Foods may also affect how well people think. A very poor diet at a young age may harm brain cells forever. Children who eat well-balanced meals do better in school. It's smart to treat your brain to good food every day!

GLOSSARY

abusing (uh BYOOZ ing) — using too much of something such as alcohol or drugs

brain cells (BRAYN SELZ) — tiny pieces that make up the brain and send signals to nerves in the body

chemicals (KEM i kulz) — stuff, such as endorphins, released in the body and used when needed

cortex (KAWR TEKS) — the gray and wrinkled outer layer of the brain

endorphins (en DAWR finz) — natural painkillers sent by the brain

liquid (LIK wid) — something that flows like water; a fluid

mind (MYND) — the part of the brain that thinks

nutrients (NOO tree ents) — good parts of foods that fuel the body

paralyzed (PAIR uh lyzd) — unable to move

spinal cord (SPY nul KORD) — a thick rope of nerves inside the spine that relays signals to and from the brain

INDEX

FURTHER READING:

Find out more about Bodyworks with these helpful books and information sites:

• Walker, Richard. *The Children's Atlas of the Human Body.* Brookfield, Connecticut: The Millbrook Press, 1994.
• Miller, Jonathan, and David Pelham. *The Human Body: The Classic Three-Dimensional Book.* New York: Penguin Books, 1983.
• Williams, Dr. Frances. *Inside Guides: Human Body.* New York: DK Publishing, 1997.

On The World Wide Web
• www.spinalcord.org. © National Spinal Cord Injury Association, 1995-1996.

On CD-ROM
• *The Family Doctor,* 3rd Edition. Edited by Allan H. Bruckheim, M.D. © Creative Multimedia, 1993-1994.